I0843435

Happy Me!
I'm Symptom Free!

Tips and Tools to Overcome
Autoimmune and Other
Chronic Conditions

Mary Ann Camarillo

Happy Me! I'm Symptom Free!

Tips and Tools to Overcome Autoimmune
and Other Chronic Conditions

The content of this book is for general instruction only. Each person's
physical, emotional, and spiritual condition is unique. The instruction
in this book is not intended to replace or interrupt the reader's
relationship with a physician or other professional. Please consult
your doctor for matters pertaining to your specific health and diet.

Printed by CreateSpace

www.createspace.com

ISBN-10: 1727492854
ISBN-13: 978-1727492859

Library of Congress Control Number: 2018912457

Printed in the United States of America

Dedication

To my husband, Al:
You're my hero, my rock, and my best friend.
Thanks for your unfailing love and support.

Acknowledgments

To Dr. Tom Matteucci of Equinox Naturopathic Medicine: Thank you for launching me on my healing journey and for your guidance along the way.

To my friend and colleague, Anita Winter: Thank you for your encouragement over the years and for sharing your editing prowess in the creation of this book.

Contents

Introduction

I had been suffering from multiple food allergies and mysterious unexplained rashes and swelling for almost ten years. Up to this point I had seen a number of doctors who all attributed my recurrent rashes to allergies, but the allergy medications did little to combat my worsening rashes and swelling.

Then in the spring of 2014 I attended a conference in San Diego, California where I first heard about gluten sensitivity and its effect on the gut. At the same time I was introduced to the term leaky gut and learned of its association with allergies and inflammation.

What I heard at that conference changed my life! It gave me hope for healing and happiness! I felt empowered to take control of my own health. I got the name of a local naturopathic doctor and quickly contacted him. At my very first visit he recommended that I eat a whole foods diet. I'm embarrassed to admit this, but at the time I literally thought that meant that I had to buy all my groceries from Whole Foods Market! Nevertheless, I was ready to take steps to transform my health. So, I went shopping the very next day and began making changes to my diet then later to my lifestyle as well.

Since I embarked on my healing journey I've often felt discouraged, misunderstood, and alone in my struggles. I've had my share of successes and setbacks, but through it all I've found the strength to persevere. I wrote this book to offer support and encouragement to all who are struggling with an autoimmune or other chronic inflammatory condition.

Throughout this book I share the tips and tools that I learned on my journey to heal my own chronic health issues. I offer simple tips and action steps to help you make small, progressive, sustainable changes so you too can enjoy greater health and happiness. Every moment is precious so get started today. The sooner you start, the sooner you'll be living a life filled with hope, healing, and happiness.

1

My Story

"I do believe in the old saying, 'What does not kill you makes you stronger.' Our experiences, good and bad, make us who we are. By overcoming difficulties, we gain strength and maturity."

Angelina Jolie

Just as no two people are exactly alike, no two stories are the same. For years I struggled with chronic health issues before finally being diagnosed with Sjogren's Syndrome, an autoimmune disease. I share the story of my own health challenges to offer hope to all who are dealing with autoimmune conditions or chronic health issues of any kind. As my story demonstrates, with patience and perseverance you can reclaim your health by making conscious, informed diet and lifestyle changes.

For most of my life I've had health problems. Since the age of five I suffered from recurring bladder infections and was given countless rounds of antibiotics over the course of my childhood. In addition, I often experienced painful stomachaches, the cause of which was never specifically determined, but was largely attributed to allergies.

These same health issues continued to plague me into adulthood, and in fact, worsened, leaving me feeling sicker and more fatigued with each passing year. My stomachaches were increasingly accompanied with severe gas and bloating and eventually with repeated bouts of diarrhea and constipation as well, which often lasted for days. The bladder infections became more frequent over time and there came a point when I started experiencing allergic reactions to a greater number of antibiotics.

As time went by I was becoming increasingly worried about my health and knew in my heart that something was just not right. However, I couldn't get any answers from my doctor, or any of the number of conventional medicine doctors that I consulted with over the years. Each time I would visit a doctor he or she would give me a physical exam, run some blood work, and tell me that I was in good health. But the problem was, that I knew I wasn't.

Just when I thought it couldn't get much worse, I started getting painful, itchy, red, swollen rashes on different parts of my body. At first, appearing when I was lightly hit or bumped, then as time went on the rashes began to develop on various parts of my body in response to light pressure from clothing or personal accessories, like a purse. Eventually it got so bad that the rashes and swelling spread to my face. On many occasions I would wake up with a swollen lip or redness and swelling around one or both of my eyes. And not only was the rash painful and itchy, but the swelling was so intense that it was literally disfiguring.

I will never forget the first time my lip swelled up. I had just started my dream job as a third grade teacher and I was teaching my students about adjectives. The students were completing an activity for which they were asked to use an adjective to describe something in the room. One student used the word "grotesque" to describe my face. I'm certain that she had no idea how hurtful her word choice was to me at the time. But nevertheless, that is exactly how I have felt each and every time I've suffered from one of my red, swollen rashes, especially when they have appeared on my face.

Because the swelling of my lip was so severe, it warranted another trip to my doctor's office. After examining me he ran some blood tests for lupus and rheumatoid arthritis, which thankfully came back negative. However, while I still had no real answers as to the nature of my problem, I was given a big clue. The blood tests showed that I had high levels of inflammation in my body. While this information meant little to me at the time, it proved to be vitally important in the coming years.

As questions still remained around the source of my rashes and swelling I was referred to an allergist who ran additional blood tests to check for food and environmental allergies. Interestingly, while the blood tests confirmed that I had several environmental allergies, no food allergies were identified. So I was sent on my way with orders to take antihistamine medication everyday. I've never been a big "pill person" but I acquiesced in hopes of alleviating my symptoms. And for a period of about four years, I experienced fewer rashes. Then there came a point when the medication seemed to be less effective, so out of frustration

I returned to the allergist to schedule a skin test, which I was told was a more sensitive method of identifying food allergies.

By this time my rashes and swelling were increasingly becoming more and more out of control. On the day of my skin test, both my arms were red and swollen to twice their normal size from my shoulders down to my wrists. More than ever, I was hoping to get some answers that might help me address the hidden allergies that had been plaguing me for so long. Well, you can only imagine my disappointment when the nurse took one look at me and said that the skin test would have to be rescheduled. Upon hearing this I literally broke down in tears and practically begged her to consult with the doctor before dismissing me. After examining me and talking with me, and hearing the desperation in my voice, the doctor agreed to perform the skin allergy test on my back instead of my arms as originally planned.

The test results were shocking to say the least. My skin reacted to every single food. The test results indicated that I was highly allergic to several foods, including some common foods that I had been eating regularly since childhood, foods like beef, potatoes, and eggs. How could this be? I didn't understand how this could be possible. And while the allergist tried to be reassuring and encouraging, I left her office that day feeling uneasy and knowing in my heart that my life would never be the same.

I knew that I had to make some major dietary changes in order to eliminate the offending allergens, particularly in regard to eggs. It wasn't too difficult to take beef and potatoes off the menu, but to my dismay I discovered that many of the processed foods that I enjoyed contained eggs. That meant that most store-bought baked goods were off limits, as well as the ranch dressing that I frequently used to drown my salads. Nevertheless, I adapted fairly quickly to my new diet and the rashes and swelling that I had been experiencing disappeared. However, the reprieve from my symptoms was short-lived, lasting only a few months. To say that I was discouraged at that point would be a gross understatement. I felt like my body was betraying me and every food that I ate became suspect. I no longer had any faith in the conventional doctors that had been caring for me so I decided to go it alone.

For three years I tried to manage my symptoms by being more mindful of my food choices, including experimenting with a gluten-free diet and taking antihistamines as needed. I certainly didn't want to live this way, if you can call it living. I prayed everyday for God's help and healing. I was thankful for the love and support of my husband and friends, but I still felt so very alone in my struggles around food. Then one day, completely out of the blue, I received a copy of *Living Without* magazine and it propelled me onto the healing journey that I am still on today.

Through the pages of *Living Without* magazine I was inspired to experiment with new recipes, and more importantly, I realized that I was not alone. I was part of a community of people suffering from allergies and food sensitivities. And as luck would have it, I saw an advertisement for the Gluten Free Food Allergy Fest that was scheduled to take place in San Diego in a few short weeks. My husband convinced me to go to the conference and for that I will always be grateful because what I learned that weekend was life-changing for me.

At the conference I attended a workshop presented by Dr. Tom O'Bryan. As he spoke about leaky gut and its association with allergies a light bulb went on in my head. I wondered, "Could a leaky gut be the root cause of my allergies?" The more I heard, the more I was convinced that I was suffering from a leaky gut. I felt instantly empowered by the prospect of healing my leaky gut and thereby eliminating my chronic allergy symptoms. Before leaving the conference I got the name of a local naturopathic doctor, Dr. Tom Matteucci.

Dr. Tom was nothing like the conventional doctors that I had previously worked with. Unlike the other doctors that I had been seeing, Dr. Tom practiced a holistic approach to healing that included diet and lifestyle changes. Instead of pills, Dr. Tom prescribed a healthy whole foods diet and helped me transition to eating an anti-inflammatory diet – starting with the elimination of gluten, dairy, and soy. Since I had already begun experimenting with a gluten-free diet that part wasn't too bad, but I resisted the idea of giving up my beloved dairy, especially cheese. It was difficult, but I eventually kicked my dairy habit. Soy was never a big part of my diet so that wasn't too hard to eliminate either. And this was just the beginning. Over time I would be forced to remove an ever-increasing number of foods from my diet in order to help my body heal.

Almost immediately I felt more energized than I had in years and the chronic bladder infections that had plagued me since childhood almost completely disappeared. However, while the frequency and intensity of my rashes diminished, they did not disappear entirely. After further testing it was determined that I had Sjogren's Syndrome, an autoimmune disease, as well as additional food sensitivities to foods that I ate on a daily basis. Again I adapted my diet to exclude the offending foods, spending hours each week scouring cookbooks and the Internet for recipes that might come close to accommodating me and cooking a whole lot more. In all honesty, I have to give my husband, Al, credit here for all the hours he's spent cooking with and for me over the last few years. Thankfully as time went by it became easier and easier to prepare meals and modify recipes that I had previously enjoyed.

But just when I thought it couldn't get any harder, I set out to eliminate all the added sugars from my diet as Dr. Tom had encouraged me to do from the start. This proved to be the greatest challenge of all, and my many failures in this endeavor left me feeling guilty and powerless. I had to come to terms with and acknowledge that I was addicted to sugar, in all its sweet and delicious forms. It's taken some time, but I've made great progress in conquering my sugar cravings. Nevertheless, it's still hard to resist a box of See's candy or to say no to a gluten-free treat of any kind. However, I've learned to appreciate a wider variety of whole foods and to acknowledge the emotions that often drove my poor food choices.

In addition to the dietary changes that I made to support my health, I implemented lifestyle changes that were equally, and in some cases, more important for my healing to take place. Like so many people, I was tired, stressed, and overscheduled on a daily basis. I had to slow down and give my body time to heal. It seems so basic, but I literally had to learn to breathe so I could release stress and bring my body to a calmer, more secure state. In addition, I committed myself to doing thirty minutes of gentle exercise each day and adjusted my schedule to allow for a minimum of seven hours of sleep each night. Together, the diet and lifestyle changes that I adopted on my healing journey helped me to resolve my chronic health issues and their accompanying physical symptoms. And may I add, that as difficult as it was to make some of these changes happen, it was well worth it. I look and feel better than I have in years!

2

Why am I Sick?

*"Life is not always easy to live, but the opportunity
to do so is a blessing beyond comprehension. In the
process of living, we will face struggles, many of which
will cause us to suffer and to experience pain."*

L. Lionel Kendrick

If you are anything like me, you've probably asked yourself this question, "Why am I sick?" While I can't answer this question for you, I have gained some powerful insights from my research into the field of functional medicine on the root causes of autoimmune and other chronic inflammatory diseases, which can help guide you in finding your own answers.

In order to understand how these diseases develop, you need to be aware of three important factors: genetics, environmental exposure, and a more recently recognized factor called leaky gut. First, you need to recognize that you are a rare flower and your body's unique genetic makeup may make you vulnerable to certain diseases or conditions. This concept is known as genetic susceptibility. The second factor, environmental exposure, refers to all the things that you come in contact with in the environment, such as foods, medicines, and chemicals, and is strongly influenced by your lifestyle. Lastly, leaky gut, also known as intestinal permeability, is the process whereby the normally tight junctions in the small intestine, or gut as it is often referred to, become inflamed and crack open, creating large holes in the lining of the small intestine.

While genetics does play a part, there are a number of environmental factors that can increase your likelihood of developing a leaky gut. New research suggests that the very food we eat, the standard American diet, which is high in sugar and saturated fat and contains little fiber, may contribute to the development of leaky gut. A connection has also been made to stress and heavy alcohol use.[1] In addition, many doctors warn that toxic chemicals found in our food, environment, medications, such as antibiotics, and even the gluten in our breads and cereals can potentially lead to a leaky gut.

Over time, having a leaky gut, with its associated increased intestinal permeability, leads to chronic inflammation, which in turn is responsible for many of the diseases that we suffer from today. Doctors have long recognized that leaky gut is linked to celiac disease, Crohn's disease, and irritable bowel syndrome (IBS). New research suggests that leaky gut may also be tied in with other autoimmune diseases, such as lupus, type 1 diabetes, multiple sclerosis, as well as chronic fatigue syndrome, fibromyalgia, arthritis, allergies, asthma, acne, obesity, and mental illness.[2] And there is increasing evidence that chronic inflammation may be the underlying cause of coronary artery disease, diabetes, cancer, and even Alzheimer's disease. [3]

Now that you're familiar with some of the factors that promote autoimmune and other chronic inflammatory diseases, I have some good news for you. You can fix your leaky gut and reduce the amount of inflammation in your body. And when you do this, your body will begin to heal and your symptoms will improve. All you have to do is take action in making important dietary and lifestyle changes. In the chapters that follow I will share the tips and tools that I used to heal my body so you too can embark on your own healing journey.

3
What Do I Do Now?

"Start by doing what's necessary; then do what's possible; and suddenly you are doing the impossible."

St. Francis of Assisi

Once you've come to terms with the true state of your health and acknowledge that you need to take action to improve your health, you must wholeheartedly commit to caring for yourself as much as you do for your loved ones. This entails practicing self-care, getting support from your family and friends, receiving care from a doctor that you trust, and working to establish greater balance in your life.

Strive for a State of Balance

You're busy each day just trying to fulfill all your various responsibilities, juggling work, home, and family responsibilities, and at the end of the day there is no time left for you. Does this scenario sound familiar? I can definitely relate. My life followed this pattern for years and years until I got so sick and tired that I just couldn't do it anymore. You and I aren't robots. We're not designed to go through life this way. It's not healthy, as I discovered firsthand, and at some point it must stop. You need to make time each day to nurture yourself: mind, body, and spirit, and to nurture your relationships as well if you are ever going to be truly healthy and happy.

On my healing journey I was forced to take stock of my life and to make important changes. I began working towards living a more balanced life. Then while studying at the Institute for Integrative Nutrition® I learned about the Circle of Life. It has proven to be an incredibly useful tool in helping me to assess different areas in my life and to achieve greater balance and satisfaction, and it can help you to do the same. Simply complete the Circle of Life as directed. First select an area that you want to improve in and commit to one or two small action steps each week until you are feeling more balanced and satisfied with that area of your life. For example, action steps that you might want to take to improve your health could be to soak your feet in warm water with Epsom salts or meditate for five to ten minutes at the end of the day. It's absolutely worth your time and effort, and you will be amazed at how even small action steps such as these can make a big difference in your health and happiness over time.

Circle of Life

The Institute for Integrative Nutrition® (IIN®) teaches
a number of dietary theories and concepts. The Circle
of Life, pictured below, is a diagram IIN® provides
to help people identify imbalances in their lives.

To complete your Circle of Life, place a dot inside
each "pie slice" to indicate your level of satisfaction
for each area. A dot toward the center indicates
dissatisfaction, and a dot toward the periphery indicates
satisfaction. For example, if your social life feels rich
and fulfilling, place a dot somewhere toward the outer
edge of the circle inside of the Social Life area.

Then, connect the dots to see which areas of
your life you are satisfied with, and which
areas you need to nurture more.

© Integrative Nutrition Inc. | Integrative Nutrition Inc.
does not endorse the content contained in this book

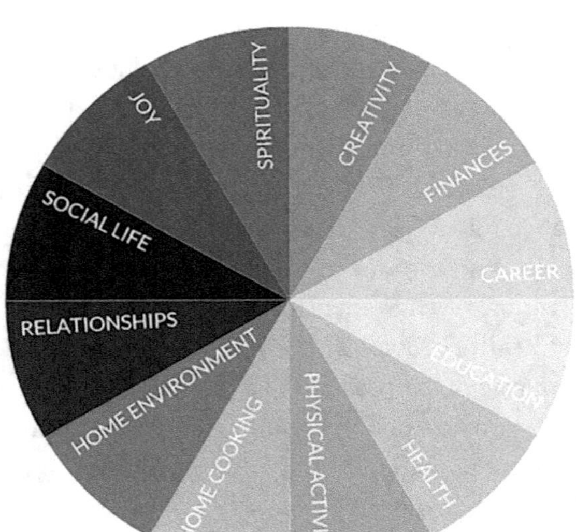

Partner with a Doctor

You have many choices when it comes to medical care and you'll want to make an informed decision on which path to take. Some approaches are: conventional medicine, alternative medicine, integrative medicine, a combination of the two approaches, and functional medicine. If you're reading this book with a diagnosis in hand you're already familiar with the conventional medicine approach, often referred to as Western or mainstream medicine. In this approach healthcare professionals, such as medical doctors, nurses, and pharmacists, address and treat symptoms predominantly with the use of drugs, radiation, or surgery. The majority of doctors seen practice conventional medicine and are primarily focused on identifying and managing diseases by alleviating patients' symptoms, thereby helping them to feel better. Conventional medicine does a pretty good job of helping people manage their diseases with prescription and over-the-counter drugs, but what it doesn't do particularly well is identify and address the root cause of their health problems. This is why so many people, including myself, turn to alternative medicine in search of real healing instead of undergoing treatments that just mask their symptoms, without really addressing the underlying health problem responsible.

The dictionary defines alternative medicine as "any range of medical therapies that are not regarded as orthodox by the medical profession". It is given the name alternative medicine because it is often used instead of conventional medicine. There are many forms of alternative medicine, but the more traditional forms include acupuncture, homeopathy, naturopathy, chiropractic medicine, Ayurveda, Chinese or oriental medicine, and a variety of energy therapies. Many of these forms of alternative medicine utilize different dietary and herbal therapies, breathing techniques, and various types of body movement, manipulation, or massage therapies. While these therapies differ from one another in their approaches, most forms of alternative medicine work to heal the mind and the body as an integrated system. The goal of alternative medicine is to bring the parts of the body back into balance naturally so the body can heal itself. It is this aspect of alternative medicine that attracts so many people who are looking to get to a better state of health without the use of powerful and often dangerous drugs or invasive surgeries.

Integrative medicine strives to combine the best of both worlds. It pairs conventional medicine with alternative medicine, often referred to as complimentary medicine when used in conjunction with conventional medical approaches. This approach considers the needs of the mind, body, and spirit, providing a more holistic approach to healing. The goal of integrative medicine is to design a personalized health plan using the most effective and least invasive treatments offered in conventional medicine in combination with proven complementary and alternative medicine (CAM) approaches. Integrative medicine is also a distinct medical specialty, where you can find doctors who are trained and board-certified.

Functional medicine is defined as "medical practice or treatments that focus on optimal functioning of the body and its organs, usually involving systems of holistic or alternative medicine." At first glance functional medicine may easily be confused with integrative medicine, but they operate in completely different ways. Both integrative and functional medicine ascribe to a holistic model of medicine that is geared to treating the whole person. However, functional medicine strives to identify the underlying cause of disease as opposed to simply creating a treatment plan, as we find with integrative medicine. In addition, most functional medicine treatment plans involve significant lifestyle changes to promote healing and overall wellness.

At this point, whether you have a specific diagnosis or not, I can't stress enough how important it is to listen to your body instead of ignoring possible warning signs and symptoms. When you do this and decide you are ready to enlist the help of a medical professional, you'll want to consider which of these approaches: conventional, alternative, integrative, or functional medicine, best suits your needs and is most closely aligned with your core values. This is a deeply personal decision that only you can make. The best advice I can offer is simply to trust your gut.

4

Food and Its Healing Power

"Your diet is a bank account. Good food choices are good investments."

Bethenny Frankel

While inflammation in the body can be a powerful tool in helping you to heal from illness or injury, too much inflammation over a long period of time becomes a destructive force. Think of this chronic inflammation as a raging fire that damages the very cells that it is designed to protect. It is through this process that autoimmune and other chronic inflammatory diseases are initiated and after a period of time, during which a significant amount of damage has been done to your body's cells, you begin to experience physical symptoms. An anti-inflammatory diet is one of the best ways to eliminate the symptoms associated with these diseases. There are two types of anti-inflammatory diets that I'd like to introduce you to: the Anti-Inflammatory diet and the Autoimmune Protocol Diet (AIP).

Anti-Inflammatory Diet

The anti-inflammatory diet is made up of mostly nutrient-dense whole plant foods. While there are many versions of the anti-inflammatory diet, with slight variations among them, the table that follows provides a basic picture. [4]

Foods to Eat	**Foods to Avoid**
Fruits and vegetables	Sugar and artificial sweeteners
Gluten-free whole grains	Fried and processed foods
Legumes	Foods containing wheat or gluten
Tree nuts	Vegetable oils, shortening, and margarine
Extra virgin olive oil	Excess alcohol and carbohydrates
Herbs and spices	
Wild-caught deep-sea fish	

It's best to choose from a variety of fruits and vegetables, because each color carries with it its own unique composition of vitamins, minerals, and other essential nutrients. With that being said, dark leafy greens and cruciferous vegetables, like broccoli and cabbage are especially good choices because they contain substances that protect our cells and help to prevent cancer. Legumes, such as soy, peas, beans, and lentils are great sources of protein and fiber. However, it is best to rinse and soak dry beans for 48-72 hours and cook them slowly in order to make them easier to digest. And while peanuts are part of the legume family, they contain naturally occurring molds, which can increase inflammation, and are therefore not included in an anti-inflammatory diet. However, tree nuts, such as almonds, walnuts, and cashews are included and they are great for snacking. Herbs and spices are great for infusing delicious flavor into your recipes, and I especially like turmeric because it has powerful anti-inflammatory properties. Cinnamon is another favorite spice of mine because it has a bit of a sweet taste and helps stave off sugar cravings while offering some anti-inflammatory benefits as well. But my advice to you is to experiment with different herbs and spices and see which ones most appeal to your taste buds.

For the benefit of those not yet familiar with the term, let's talk a little about gluten. Gluten is the general name of a family of proteins found in grains like wheat, rye, and barley. There are several different forms of wheat, each with its own distinct name, such as spelt and kamut. Some studies have demonstrated a link between gluten and leaky gut in certain sensitive individuals.[5] In addition, we now know that having a leaky gut leads to increased inflammation. Therefore, it is recommended that you eat gluten-free whole grains such as quinoa, basmati or brown rice, millet, amaranth, buckwheat, teff, and gluten-free oats on the anti-inflammatory diet.

Now let's take a minute to clarify what constitutes a processed food. Put simply, it is any food that has been changed from its whole, natural state. With that being said, there are different degrees of food processing that make foods more or less healthy. For example, you can purchase an apple or a piece of steak that has been cut for you; the simple act of cutting is considered a form of food processing, but it doesn't make the apple or steak any less healthy. However, foods that are highly processed, such as cookies, crackers, and chips, often have added sugars, preservatives, and fats added to enhance their taste and texture, and to prolong their shelf life. These foods are far removed from their original, natural state and should be avoided. In general, a good rule of thumb to follow is this: the shorter the list of ingredients on the bag or box, the better.

I'd like to offer you a little more insight into the foods to avoid on the anti-inflammatory diet. First, you're probably curious as to why excess alcohol is listed on the chart. Why not just eliminate alcohol completely from your diet? Well, the answer is that studies have shown that consuming red wine in moderation actually has health benefits due to the phytonutrient, resveratrol that is naturally found in red wine. It turns out that resveratrol is a very powerful compound that protects your body's cells from damage. In addition, while it is important to eat a combination of healthy fats, proteins, and carbohydrates at every meal, consuming excess carbohydrates not only raises your blood sugar more than necessary, but studies have shown that it may promote inflammation. Also, I want to offer a couple of words about caffeine and nightshade vegetables. While they are not specifically listed as foods to avoid, you may want to consider it. Caffeine can raise levels of a stress hormone known as cortisol. And since stress is linked to leaky gut, it's best to avoid caffeine as much as possible. Instead of drinking coffee, you may want to try green tea. While green tea does contain caffeine, it contains significantly lower levels of caffeine compared to coffee. Lastly, nightshade vegetables, such as tomatoes, potatoes, eggplants, and peppers can increase inflammation in some people, so you may want to eliminate nightshade vegetables for a few weeks. Then you can gradually reintroduce these foods into your diet and see how you feel.

Hopefully you've already noticed that there are a greater number of foods that you can eat versus foods that you should avoid on the basic anti-inflammatory diet. I point this out because it is easy to get caught up in your emotions around food and feel like you are being deprived in some way when you follow this diet, or any other for that matter. This type of negative thinking can get you off track and send you into bouts of emotional eating that are guaranteed to set you back. I can speak about this because it has happened to me countless times over the course of my healing journey, leaving me feeling powerless and ashamed each and every time. Instead of falling prey to these cycles of negative thinking, I encourage you to focus on the positive aspects, such as the inner healing that is taking place in your body with each bite of food, the tremendous gift of health that you are giving yourself, and the personal growth that is occurring, transforming you into a better, stronger person.

Autoimmune Protocol Diet

The autoimmune protocol diet (AIP) is a paleo version of the anti-inflammatory diet that is more specifically designed for people suffering from autoimmune conditions. Like the anti-inflammatory diet, there are several versions of the AIP diet that differ slightly from one another. In general, the AIP diet is an elimination diet that mainly consists of meats and vegetables. The table below lists the foods that you should eat and those that you should avoid on the autoimmune protocol diet.[6]

Foods to Eat	Foods to Avoid
Grass-fed, organic meats and wild-caught fish	All grains
Vegetables, all except nightshades	All legumes, including soy, beans, and peanuts
Sweet potatoes (not part of the nightshade family:)	All dairy products, including butter and ghee
Fruit (in limited amounts)	Sugars and artificial sweeteners
Fermented foods, such as kombucha, non-dairy kefir, sauerkraut	Processed foods
Avocado, olive, and coconut oil	Vegetable oils
Vinegars, including balsamic, red wine, and apple cider vinegar	Eggs
Organic raw honey and pure maple syrup (in small amounts)	Nuts and seeds, including coffee, chocolate, and spices derived from seeds

Non-seed herbs, such as basil and oregano	Nightshade vegetables
Coconut products, such as coconut milk, coconut butter, and shredded coconut	Food additives, like emulsifiers and thickeners
Bone broth	Alcohol
Green tea	NSAIDS (Non-steroidal, anti-inflammatory drugs, like aspirin, ibuprofen, naproxen)

* The AIP diet is a powerful tool to help you identify which foods your body is sensitive to and which foods work best for you.

As you can see, the AIP diet is much more restrictive than the basic anti-inflammatory diet. It is an elimination diet that is designed to help heal a leaky gut and reset your immune system by removing all the foods that your body may be sensitive to and that may be contributing to your leaky gut, ultimately increasing inflammation. Not only that, but the AIP diet incorporates gut-healing bone broth into your diet as well as fermented foods that are full of natural probiotics that support a healthy digestive system.

By now you may be wondering how you can ever stick to the AIP diet. Well, the good news is that you don't need to stick to it forever. Generally you follow the diet for four weeks, and then gradually add healthy foods that you excluded back into your diet. It's best to reintroduce one new food every two or three days while monitoring your reactions each day and noting them in a food journal. If you do experience any type of reaction, then you should eliminate that food from your diet completely and wait until your reaction clears up before adding another new food and starting the process all over again. While following the AIP diet is not easy and the process of reintroducing foods back into your diet is slow and a bit tedious, it is well worth it to gain powerful insight into the foods that are best for your body.

The Choice is Up to You

When it comes to food I really like to have choices. With that being said, both the basic anti-inflammatory diet and the autoimmune protocol diet are both good choices for decreasing inflammation in the body. I have followed both these diets at different times and have experienced their healing benefits, specifically with the reduction in frequency and severity of my symptoms. The AIP diet was undoubtedly much harder to follow during the four week elimination phase, and I had an especially hard time giving up nuts, seeds, and grains, but once I was able to incorporate some of these favorites back into my diet, it was much easier to maintain my healthy eating habits. The basic anti-inflammatory diet, being much less restrictive, was most definitely easier to follow over the long term. Nevertheless, I have to say that I modified it to include small amounts of animal protein, such as grass-fed beef and organic poultry.

5
Listen to Your Body

"When you are balanced and when you listen and attend to the needs of your body, mind, and spirit, your natural beauty comes out."
Christy Turlington

The best advice that I can give you as you embark on a new chapter in your healing journey is to listen to your body. Your body knows intuitively what it needs and when you give it what it needs, your body will return the favor, giving you a greater sense of overall wellness. Your sleep, energy, mood, and focus will improve and if you've been experiencing other physical symptoms they will start to subside. I say this with confidence because that is exactly what happened to me and to others with whom I've mentored in my health coaching practice.

Keep a Food/Wellness Journal

As you become more skilled at listening to your body's subtle messages it is absolutely essential that you keep a food journal, or what I like to call, a wellness journal. Every day you will record the following information in your wellness journal:

1. Foods eaten and approximate quantity
2. Activities engaged in
3. Intense emotions or feelings (if applicable)
4. Any symptoms/reactions experienced
5. Time associated with any reactions
6. Rating of the intensity of any reactions on a scale of 1-10 (with 1 being least and 10 being most intense)

Refer to the sample wellness journal that follows to get an idea of how to set it up or download a copy of the wellness journal template from my health coaching website at www.hopeforhealingandhappiness.com.

Date	Foods / Feelings / Activities	Reactions, if any / (Rating)	Time
8/1	Breakfast: Scrambled egg with spinach		
	Lunch: Chicken salad with avocado dressing		

	Emotions: Stressed at work over a deadline	Headache (4)	2pm
	Snack: apple		
	Dinner: Turkey Meatloaf with mashed sweet potatoes		
	Activity: Walked the dog		

Let's take a minute to explore some of the reactions that should be included in your wellness journal. Of course you're going to include major symptoms like pain, swelling, hives, and headaches. However, there are a whole host of subtle, less intense reactions that you should acknowledge, such as sweating, runny nose, itching, indigestion, dizziness, or irritability, just to name a few. It may sound crazy, but your body uses these and countless other ways to communicate with you each and every day. As for myself, in addition to the major symptoms that I experienced over the years: the stomach aches, gas and bloating, diarrhea, constipation, and eventually the swollen rashes, there were many seemingly unimportant clues that I ignored such as, frequent canker sores, itching sensations in my ears, leg cramps at night, and swollen fingers upon waking each morning.

If I had only listened to my body then and acknowledged that there was a problem, I could have addressed it and spared myself years of suffering, but I didn't know then what

I know now. Namely, if you are knowingly or unknowingly eating foods that you are sensitive or allergic to, engaging in activities that don't support you, or harboring negative emotions or unhealthy levels of stress, your body will send subtle and not so subtle SOS signals and continue sending them out until you listen and make some lifestyle changes. Now is the time to tune in to your body and learn to recognize and decode the messages that it is sending out. This is where the wellness journal comes in. It is such a powerful tool in helping you to identify patterns and to zone in on the foods, feelings, and activities that may or may not be supporting your optimal health and happiness at this time.

As you complete your wellness journal each day, noting the foods, emotions, and activities that are part of your daily life and recording any symptoms or reactions that you experience, it is important to consider the timing associated with any reactions that you may be having. Some reactions may be immediately felt, while others could take hours or even days to appear. I know for me personally, some reactions took almost a week to occur. I believe that the timing just depends on your body and the level of inflammation that you have at specific times. Therefore, I recommend noting the time that you first notice a reaction. Lastly, be conscious of the intensity and severity of any reactions and rate the level of intensity next to each reaction listed in your wellness journal. It is interesting to note here that when I looked at the intensity of my rashes and swelling over time, I realized that the more severe reactions not only occurred when I was exposed to foods that I was allergic or highly sensitive to, but also when I was experiencing higher levels of stress. The practice of keeping a wellness journal really helped me to listen more closely to my body and to honor it by responding to its unique needs.

Hidden Allergies and Food Sensitivities

If you're faithfully following an anti-inflammatory diet and making a conscious and consistent effort to reduce your stress levels, you will begin to notice small improvements to your health, such as a reduction in the frequency and intensity of your symptoms, better focus, memory, and mood, as well as increased energy. While it will take some time for any major, lasting changes to take place, you should start to feel better in a matter of days or weeks. If you aren't seeing any progress after a few weeks, hidden allergies and food sensitivities may be to blame.

As I learned on my healing journey, leaky gut can contribute to the development of food allergies and sensitivities. Even if you haven't experienced any symptoms specifically attributable to allergies, you may indeed have food sensitivities that are causing inflammation and interfering with the healing process. As for myself, testing revealed that not only did I have undiagnosed allergies, but also that I was highly sensitive to a number of seemingly healthy foods, including broccoli, string beans, and most surprisingly, garlic. Therefore, if you are not able to pinpoint the source of your allergies, or most likely food sensitivities, through your use of the Wellness Journal, I would strongly recommend that you consult with your doctor about getting tested for allergies and food sensitivities.

6

Knowledge is Power

"I feel like knowledge is power: If you know how to take care of yourself, you can be a better version of yourself."
Miranda Kerr

A Word About Water

Our bodies are made up mostly of water and we all know how essential water is to our very existence, but you may not be aware of some of the wonderful health benefits that water offers. First and foremost, water helps remove wastes and toxins from our bodies, aids in digestion, and can prevent constipation. Drinking water shortly before meals also helps to satiate you, making you feel full so you can eat less and maintain a healthy weight. In addition, water can prevent and relieve muscle cramps and some types of headaches. Staying hydrated also helps to boost energy, to optimize brain function, and it helps your skin look younger at the same time.

In order to take advantage of all the benefits that water has to offer, you need to be drinking an adequate amount of water each day. A simple rule of thumb that I use to guide my daily water consumption is to drink half my body weight in ounces of water each day. For example, if you weigh 140 lbs., you would need to drink about 70 ounces of water per day. However, the exact amount of water that you need each day depends on your age and gender, as well as other factors such as the weather, your activity level, and your overall health. Therefore, I encourage you to experiment and determine for yourself what amount of water works best for you and your body.

Simple Tips:

- Drink one to two glasses of water within thirty minutes of waking in the morning.
- Drink a glass of water after every trip to the bathroom.
- Set the timer on your phone to remind you to drink some water every hour.
- Add 1 TBSP fresh-squeezed lemon juice to a cup of warm water and drink every morning to help detox your liver.
- Add 1 TBSP of organic, unfiltered, apple cider vinegar to a half cup of water. Drink this mixture a few minutes before each meal to help your digestion and to make you feel more satiated.

> • To help curb sugar cravings when they arise, drink a glass of water. Add a splash of lemon juice or apple cider vinegar if you like.

Chemicals in Our Food Supply

In addition to the chemical stabilizers and preservatives that are often found in processed food, most conventionally produced meat and produce sold in the United States today contain chemicals in various forms as well. Antibiotics are routinely used to produce conventionally raised beef, poultry, pork, and farm-raised fish. [7]

In addition to antibiotics, scientists have found traces of other drugs, such as antidepressants and antifungal medications in samples of beef, pork, and poultry.[8] Most cattle and sheep are also given hormones to facilitate growth and meat production. In addition, ractopamine is a chemical feed additive that is commonly given to pigs, and to some cattle and turkeys as well, to promote growth and increase lean muscle mass.[9] In addition, the conventionally grown produce that we buy at the grocery store can contain any number of different chemicals in the form of pesticides and herbicides which are harmful not only to insects and plants, but also to people and other animals. While pesticides are useful for controlling a variety of unwanted pests, and herbicides are very effective at killing weeds, these chemicals can contaminate the land, the water, the air, and the very food we eat.

Despite the fact that the use of these chemical substances is perfectly legal according to the United States Food and

Drug Administration, there is some scientific evidence linking these chemicals to negative health consequences, including cancer. Therefore, a whole host of medical practitioners, such as functional medicine doctors and naturopaths, recommend that you limit your consumption of foods containing these chemicals. So in keeping with their recommendations you should purchase grass-fed or organic meats and wild-caught fish whenever possible. As far as produce is concerned, the same recommendation applies. It is generally best to eat organic fruits and vegetables as opposed to their conventionally grown counterparts. Not only do organic fruits and vegetables taste better, but some studies have also shown that they contain higher levels of antioxidants, which are naturally occurring compounds that protect our cells from damage.

The Dirty Dozen and The Clean Fifteen

Considering all the benefits that organic foods have to offer, why doesn't everyone eat strictly organic? In a word, cost. Organic meats and produce are significantly more expensive to buy, and let's face it: Most of us are living on a budget that doesn't afford us the luxury of eating all organically grown foods. Thankfully for all of us the Environmental Working Group (EWG) is here to help.

The EWG is a non-profit organization that works to protect our environment and our health. This group does a lot of research and community outreach to educate people on public health issues. One example of this is EWG's annual "Shopper's Guide to Pesticides in Produce". (https://www.ewg.org/foodnews) In this guide the EWG details the most contaminated produce in its "Dirty Dozen" list and the safest conventional produce in its "Clean Fifteen" list. Using these lists will allow you to make more informed decisions around which organic foods are really worth splurging on and which ones aren't worth spending the extra money.

Check out EWG's 2018 top picks in each category below:

<table>
<tr><td><u>Dirty Dozen</u></td><td><u>Clean Fifteen</u></td></tr>
<tr><td>Strawberries</td><td>Avocados</td></tr>
<tr><td>Spinach</td><td>Sweet Corn</td></tr>
<tr><td>Nectarines</td><td>Pineapples</td></tr>
<tr><td>Apples</td><td>Cabbages</td></tr>
<tr><td>Grapes</td><td>Onions</td></tr>
<tr><td>Peaches</td><td>Sweet Peas</td></tr>
<tr><td>Cherries</td><td>Papayas</td></tr>
<tr><td>Pears</td><td>Asparagus</td></tr>
<tr><td>Tomatoes</td><td>Mangoes</td></tr>
<tr><td>Celery</td><td>Eggplants</td></tr>
<tr><td>Potatoes</td><td>Honeydew Melons</td></tr>
<tr><td>Sweet Bell Peppers</td><td>Kiwis</td></tr>
<tr><td>Plus:</td><td>Cantaloupes</td></tr>
<tr><td>Hot Peppers</td><td>Cauliflower</td></tr>
<tr><td></td><td>Broccoli</td></tr>
</table>

Food Substitutes

When I first started following the Autoimmune Protocol Diet (AIP) I had a difficult time finding recipes that could accommodate my body's unique needs, so I began experimenting with healthy food substitutes to replace the ingredients that are commonly found in recipes with AIP-approved ingredients. In the table that follows I have listed some of my favorite go-to food substitutions that work in a variety of recipes.

Instead of:	Substitute:
1 large egg	1 TBSP ground flax or chia seed mixed with 3-4 TBSP warm water OR 4 TBSP unsweetened applesauce mixed with 1 tsp baking powder OR * 3 TBSP aquafaba (water from canned chickpeas or other legumes)
Cornstarch	Arrowroot Powder
1 cup cow's milk	1 cup coconut milk
Potatoes	Sweet Potatoes, Turnips, or Rutabagas
Parmesan Cheese	Nutritional Yeast
Spaghetti Noodles	Spiralized Zucchini or Spaghetti Squash
Flours (made of grains, nuts, or legumes)	Cassava, Tiger Nut, or Coconut Flour

Sugar	Organic Raw Honey or Pure Maple Syrup OR * Date Paste
Vegetable Oils	Olive, Avocado, or Coconut Oil
Tree Nuts (almonds, cashews, etc.)	Tiger Nuts (small root vegetables)

* Not approved for the Autoimmune Protocol Diet, but a great food substitute.

Probiotics and Prebiotics

About 100 trillion bacteria, collectively referred to as the "gut flora" or "gut microbiota", reside in your gut. The gut flora is made up of a combination of good and bad bacteria. In a healthy gut there is a healthy balance of good and bad bacteria. However, a number of factors can alter the gut flora, reducing the number of good bacteria and increasing the number of bad bacteria, causing an imbalance known as dysbiosis. In turn, this dysbiosis can cause gas and bloating and lead to a whole host of health concerns, including inflammation, insulin resistance, weight gain and obesity, inflammatory bowel disease, and colorectal cancer.[10]

Probiotics help to maintain a diverse and balanced gut flora. Probiotics are the good bacteria found in your gut, and you can take them as supplements or consume them in a variety of fermented foods, such as raw sauerkraut, kimchi, and fermented vegetables, as well as yogurt and kefir, if you can tolerate dairy. If you are up for a challenge, I would highly encourage you to experiment by making your own fermented vegetables.

While they work in a slightly different way, prebiotics also support a healthy balance of good and bad bacteria in the gut. Prebiotics are dietary fibers that can't be digested by the body, but are used instead to feed the good bacteria, helping them to work better. Prebiotics are found in a variety of foods, including whole grain oats, garlic and onions, asparagus, apples and bananas, leafy green vegetables, and my personal favorite, cocoa.

7

Harness the Power of the Mind/Body Connection

"You create your own universe as you go along."
Winston Churchill

The Power of the Mind

Our thoughts are powerful constructs shaped by our perceptions and inspired by our senses: the sights, sounds, and experiences of our daily lives. In turn our thoughts inspire our words and actions. Whether we are conscious of it or not, our thoughts influence and are influenced by our feelings and emotions, and these same thoughts can have a powerful impact on our physical body and overall sense of well-being.

To illustrate the incredible power of the mind I want to share a personal story. A few years ago I read *The Secret* by Rhonda Bryne. I was intrigued by the title and curious as to what secret the book promised to reveal. As it turned out the book was about harnessing the power of the mind to manifest positive things in your life. Shortly after reading the book I performed an experiment of sorts to prove or disprove the book's claim that whatever thoughts you turn your attention to will manifest themselves in your life. This experiment entailed focusing my mind on noticing and counting the number of butterflies that I saw over a period of several days. Now keep in mind that I was performing this little experiment during the winter months when live butterflies are hard to find even in temperate regions. However, I was utterly astonished by the number of butterflies and butterfly images that I took notice of in my immediate surroundings. It was certainly an eye-opening experience on the tremendous power of the mind.

Positive Thinking and Gratitude

Let's face it. We all experience good and bad times during the course of our lives, but we have the power to rise above our circumstances by using positive thinking. The following quote comes to mind when considering the concept of positive thinking: "I can complain because rose bushes have thorns or I can rejoice because thorn bushes have roses." Positive thinking is a way of thinking about the present that opens your mind up to seeing all the good things in your life and appreciating them. Sounds a little like gratitude doesn't it? That's because positive thinking and gratitude go hand in hand. If you turn your awareness to all the good things in your life you'll naturally feel more grateful, and vice versa, and when you show gratitude more positive things will come your way.

> Tips to Nurture Positive Thinking and Gratitude:
>
> - Speak positively at all times regardless of the situation. (Or as my mom used to say, "If you don't have anything nice to say, don't say anything at all.")
> - Acknowledge that you are blessed every day.
> - When you drink a glass of water or sit down to enjoy a meal, be thankful for having access to clean water and nourishing food.
> - At the end of each day write down 3-5 things that you are thankful for in a "Gratitude Journal".
> - If you are having a difficult day take a moment to stop, take a deep calming breath, and find something positive to celebrate, such as a happy memory, or gratitude for having a job or a loving family.

Managing Stress

Stress is the body's natural defense reaction to any change that requires a response. The body is designed to respond to these changes physically, mentally, or emotionally, and all is well and good until stress continues over prolonged periods of time. This is referred to as chronic stress, and it is neither normal nor natural. It is this chronic stress that wears down the body physically and emotionally, causing a variety of physical and emotional problems. Research confirms that chronic stress can cause or exacerbate certain diseases. This is why it is vitally important that you take steps every day to reduce stress and tension in your daily life. Some of the relaxation techniques that I found most helpful are the following:

Meditation – Many people, including myself at one time, strictly view meditation as a process in which you completely free your mind from thoughts as you sit quietly and breathe. However, meditation is an art that can take many forms, all of which allow you to be present in the moment and to focus on your body and breath. Closing your eyes also helps you to focus inward and to create a deeper awareness inside you. If you are interested in starting a meditation practice you may want to try the *Insight Timer* app for inspiration.

Mindfulness – This is actually a form of meditation. Being mindful simply involves focusing on one activity at a time and noticing the sights, sounds, smells, and tastes around you at the present time, in much the same way a young child experiences the world.

Grounding/Earthing – As the name implies, grounding is putting your body in direct contact with the ground, specifically the surface of the earth. You can ground by simply touching the earth with your skin or through the use of a commercially available grounding system. Researchers have found that grounding, when done frequently over a sustained period of time, offers health benefits, such as the reduction of pain and inflammation.[11] In light of this information you may want to consider purchasing a grounding system, but I would definitely encourage you to spend at least fifteen minutes outside barefooted each day, and either sit and meditate or walk around your yard, neighborhood, or a local park to absorb the earth's healing electrical energy.

Conscious Breathing – This activity simply entails taking deep, calming breaths to relieve tension and calm the nervous system. Throughout the day whenever you feel tension or stress building up inside, just stop and take 2-3 deep breaths in and out. One of my favorite conscious breathing exercises comes from Dr. Andrew Weil, and it is referred to as the 4-7-8 Breathing Exercise, also aptly named the Relaxing Breath. I like to do this breathing exercise in the car on my way to and from work, but you can do it any time, especially when you're feeling stressed or upset.

> The 4-7-8 Breathing Exercise:
>
> 1. Exhale loudly through your open mouth, making a "whooshing" sound as you do so.
> 2. Touch the tip of your tongue against the gum tissue behind your upper front teeth and keep it there throughout the entire exercise.
> 3. Close your mouth and inhale quietly through your nose to a count of four.
> 4. Hold your breath for a count of seven.
> 5. Exhale loudly through your open mouth for a count of eight.
> 6. Repeat steps 3-5 above three more times for a total of four breaths.

Self-Care Activities – These include any activities that bring you joy and help you to relax and to find balance in your life. Aim to do one self-care activity every day. Some examples of self-care activities:

- Take an Epsom salt bath. (my personal favorite)
- Read a favorite book or magazine.
- Sit outside and do some grounding.
- Get (or give yourself) a facial, manicure, or pedicure.
- Have lunch with a friend.
- Light a candle and meditate.
- Eat outside on the patio or in the backyard.
- Get a massage.
- Take a walk or go for a hike. (I like to take my dog with me.)
- Listen to your favorite music.
- Take a dance or yoga class.

These are just a few examples of self-care activities that I enjoy. Feel free to try some of these or find other self-care activities that you like.

Feeling and Dealing with Emotions

Emotions, in and of themselves, are neither good nor bad; they are simply ways for us to get in touch with our inner selves. However, many of us, myself included, have never really learned how to feel and deal with our emotions. As children we are often taught to suppress our emotions, or as my elder daughter poetically says, "Suck it up." However, the problem with this tactic is that the emotions that don't get acknowledged and addressed don't just disappear. They stick around, moving from our conscious mind into our subconscious mind, causing us to think, say, and do all kinds of crazy, inexplicable things. Therefore, it's important to take the time to fully process our emotions when they arise. In this way we are able to resolve any issues and release our negative emotions instead of carrying them around as emotional baggage in our subconscious suitcase.

Much of the difficulty that I have had, and that you may have experienced as well, in eliminating sugar and transitioning away from the comfort foods that have been a big part of my life since childhood, stems from the fact that I have often used food to deal with my emotions. Before I could even begin to heal my physical body I had to look inside myself and come to terms with two truths: I was an emotional eater and I was addicted to sugar. Not only could I not resist the sweet treats that seemed to call my name, but I also often ate to soothe my emotions. I turned to sugar and processed foods when I felt just about anything: happy, sad, mad, lonely, tired, you name it. It has taken some time, and is still in fact a work in progress, but I have begun to acknowledge some painful emotions: feelings of guilt, shame, fear, sadness, and loneliness. It was not until I started to address my emotional eating and sugar addiction that I was able to really stick to the anti-inflammatory diet for any extended length of time.

Hopefully your relationship with food is not as complicated as my own. Keep in mind though that food has the power to evoke powerful memories and strong emotions. Therefore, it is important to acknowledge how incredibly difficult it can be to make even small dietary changes, much less the changes necessary to completely revamp your entire daily diet in order to support your health. With that in mind, remember to be gentle with yourself and treat yourself with loving kindness and understanding, just as you would treat a young child in your care. Feelings of guilt or shame have no place on your healing journey. Take the time to acknowledge that you are only human and that you're doing the best you can.

8

Sleep and Exercise: Two Powerful Practices Not to Pass Up

"Take rest; a field that has rested gives a bountiful crop."

Ovid

In addition to eating foods that truly nourish your body, it is absolutely essential that you get optimal amounts of sleep and physical activity each day to further support the health of both your mind and body. I use the term optimal here, because each person is unique, requiring a distinct amount of sleep and physical activity to reach and maintain optimum health and wellness. While it will take some commitment and extra effort on your part, scheduling adequate time for sleep and engaging in some form of daily physical activity, are key to reaping the countless, amazing benefits of these two powerful practices.

Sleep is Healing

Sleep is so important for our physical, mental, and emotional health. Good sleep strengthens our immune system, increases energy, alertness, and even improves mood. I'm sure you're well aware of the generally accepted recommendation that adults sleep seven to nine hours each night. Why then, do most of us struggle and often fail to get enough sleep? We all have our reasons, but in my experience I've found that the two most common reasons why people don't get enough sleep stem from overscheduling or insomnia.

Overscheduling, as the name implies, refers to trying to do too much each day. I have often fallen into this trap when creating my daily to-do list. Each morning I would list all the things that I wanted to accomplish that day. However, I found myself adding items to my list as the day wore on. Then instead of completing my original short list, I found myself stressing over the remaining unfinished items on my list at the end of the day and pushing my bedtime back later and later in an attempt to finish my to-do list. Now my to-do list was complete, but I had a new problem. I wasn't getting enough hours of sleep each night because the alarm clock was still going off at its non-negotiable scheduled time. It was a vicious cycle that left me feeling tired and stressed. Clearly, any rational person could see that this method wasn't supporting my health or happiness and that change was a must. However, before I could make any meaningful and lasting change in my daily habits I had to respect the fact that there are only twenty-four hours in a day and acknowledge that I can't spend them all working. From that point on I started prioritizing my time more effectively and efficiently, allowing time for work, and just as importantly, time for me. And as a result, I'm getting the sleep I need and enjoying a happier, healthier, and more balanced life.

Scheduling Tips:

- Schedule time in your daily schedule for self-care and social activities.
- Commit and stick to a regular bedtime.
- Prioritize the items on your to-do list each day. (Moving any unfinished items to the next day.)
- Estimate the time needed and allow enough time for each activity that you have scheduled.

Insomnia, or the inability to sleep, is a big problem today affecting an increasing number of people. Typically people suffering from insomnia have trouble falling asleep or staying asleep at night. Insomnia can be caused by a variety of physical and psychological factors, such as medical conditions or medications, hormone levels, or lifestyle factors.[12] Depending on the cause, there are a number of medical and behavioral treatments that you can try to combat insomnia. If you are struggling with insomnia you may want to experiment with some of the sleep tips listed below and see how they impact your sleep.

Tips for Better Sleep:

- Keep a consistent sleep schedule by going to bed and getting up at the same time each day.
- Avoid eating heavy meals or highly processed foods for dinner.
- Sleep in a cool, comfortable, and quiet place.
- Use blackout curtains and keep your bedroom as dark as possible.
- Share any thoughts, worries or negative emotions from the day with a friend or loved one or write them down in a journal before going to bed.
- Read or meditate before bed.
- Avoid intense physical activity within one to two hours of bedtime.
- Limit liquids during the two hours prior to bedtime.
- Eat dinner three or more hours before bed.
- Watch and enjoy the beauty of the sunset.
- Turn off all electronic devices, such as computers, cell phones, TVs, etc. at least one to two hours before bed.
- Dim the lights in the house as bedtime approaches.

Sleep Diary

While studying to be a health coach at the Institute for Integrative Nutrition®, I was introduced to the concept of a sleep diary. Since that time I've learned that doctors often use sleep diaries to help diagnose sleep disorders in their patients. A sleep diary can be an incredibly useful tool that can not only help your doctor, but it can also help you to make connections and discern patterns between your daily diet and activities, and the quantity and quality of your sleep each night. If you are struggling with insomnia I strongly recommend that you keep a sleep diary and pay special attention to your activities during the evening hours leading up to bedtime. When you keep a sleep diary, even for a short period of time, you'll most likely become aware of lifestyle factors that are interfering with your sleep. For example, I kept a sleep diary for a week and found that I didn't sleep as well when I ate a heavy fat-laden meal for dinner, when I ate certain processed or sugary foods, and when I ate too late in the evening.

If you are working with a doctor to address problems with insomnia, he or she may ask you to complete a specific type of sleep diary or log. I found the following sleep diary extremely useful in helping me to determine the factors that were impacting the quantity and quality of my daily sleep. Even if you don't suffer from insomnia, this is a great exercise for those of you who are curious about how your current lifestyle may be affecting your sleep. Simply complete your sleep diary for one or two weeks and analyze your findings. You may be surprised at what you find. To get started you will need to record the following information in your sleep diary every day:

1. Total number of hours slept each day
2. Rating of the quality of my sleep (on a scale of 1-10)

3. Interruptions to my sleep (bathroom runs, environmental noises, etc.)
4. Thoughts and activities experienced shortly before bed and/or during the night
5. Food, drinks, and medications consumed during the day, noting specific medications and paying special attention to caffeine, alcohol, and foods with sugar or chemical additives
6. Am I alert and energetic upon waking and throughout the day?

Refer to the sample sleep diary that follows to get an idea of how to set it up or download a copy of the sleep diary template from my health coaching website at www.hopeforhealingandhappiness.com.

Date	# of Hours Sleep	Quality of Sleep (1-10)	# of Sleep Interruptions/ Causes	Thoughts / Activities before bed and/ or during the night	Amount of caffeine, alcohol, sugar, chemical additives and/or medications consumed	Alert and Energetic all day? (Y/N)
8/15	7	8	2 bathroom run and dog barking	Computer work until 9pm	Small amount of caffeine in tea	Yes

When keeping a sleep diary it is important to record all the information that you can, because even seemingly unimportant information can play a powerful role in helping you and your doctor to determine the factors that may be contributing to your insomnia and to effectively address those factors so you can sleep better at night.

Physical Activity

Our bodies are designed to move and daily physical activity, a.k.a. exercise, is absolutely essential to our overall health. Not only does exercise help us to stay physically fit, but it also increases our physical and mental energy. There are three main types of exercise that you should aim to do each week: cardiovascular exercise, strength training, and flexibility training. Cardiovascular exercise, also referred to as aerobic exercise, is any fast-paced exercise that gets your heart rate up and requires you to use more oxygen. Examples of cardiovascular exercise, or cardio for short, are walking, running, and bike riding. Strength training is an anaerobic form of exercise that is designed to build and maintain muscles. Flexibility training or stretching is a form of exercise that helps to lengthen muscles and to increase the range of motion of joints. Yoga is a great example of a flexibility training exercise and one of my personal favorites. Regardless of which type of exercise you choose or how long you engage in it each day, you will reap the tremendous benefits that exercise has to offer.

If you're finding it hard to exercise regularly, it is totally understandable. You lead a busy life, juggling work and family, and you don't have the time or the energy to devote to daily exercise. What's more, you may be experiencing a lot of pain or discomfort if you are currently suffering from an autoimmune disease. These are all very real and valid reasons to forego exercise. But what if I told you that just a few minutes of moderate exercise has a myriad of health benefits, including the power to boost your energy and mood, protect your memory, help you sleep better, and reduce chronic pain, [13] would your reconsider? As much as it is a challenge to schedule and commit to some form of daily physical activity, it is well worth your time and effort. We're only talking about five minutes of exercise each day, and it doesn't have to be hard or intense exercise. In fact, I've found that light to moderate intensity exercise works best for me. The best part about exercise is that absolutely anyone can do it. You don't have to go to an expensive gym everyday, just invest in a good pair of walking shoes to start. Then start! If you're looking for ideas or inspiration there are some great exercise programs on cable TV and videos online that you can check out, or you can just experiment on your own. After a period of time you may even want to increase the time and intensity of your daily exercise as your body grows stronger and healthier. When it comes to physical activity and exercise, like everything else, simply do what feels right for you.

9

Cultivate Strong Social and Spiritual Connections

Maslow's Hierarchy of Needs

As the American psychologist, Abraham Maslow outlined in his famous theory, known as Maslow's Hierarchy of Needs, all human beings have the same human needs. According to his theory, basic needs found in the lower tiers of the hierarchy must be met before addressing the needs listed in the higher tiers.[14] In contemplating Maslow's Hierarchy of Needs it is clear that you and I have a strong, basic psychological need to connect with others. Dean Ornish expressed this best when he said, "The need for connection and community is primal, as fundamental as the need for air, water, and food."

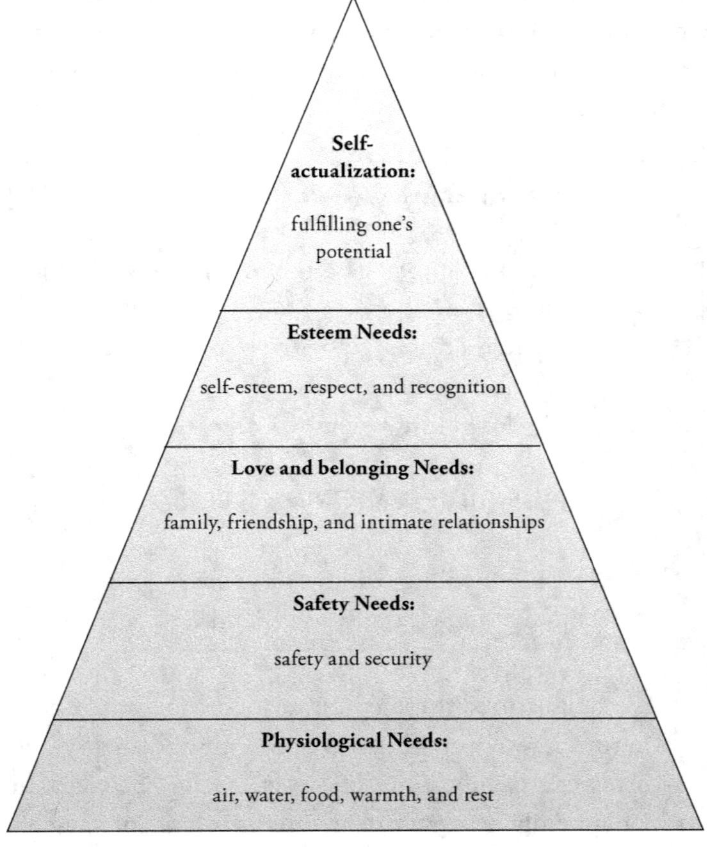

Supportive Relationships

We access the connection we need through relationships with others: family, friends, and loved ones. The people in our lives offer us fresh perspectives, help us grow, and broaden our vision. They encourage us and give us strength during difficult times and are there to celebrate our victories, large and small alike.

Tips to Strengthen Your Relationships:

- Schedule time each evening to spend with your spouse or loved one.
- Schedule a date night with your spouse or loved one once a week.
- Call close family members and friends at least once a week.
- Meet with a friend for lunch or dinner once a month.
- Be more willing to give of yourself. (Say "yes" more often to family and friends.)

We are nurtured through our relationships with others, and in turn it's important that we put time and energy into nurturing our relationships. However, during the constant rush of our daily lives, we can all too easily lose our valuable connections with others. As a case in point, think about all the friends that you've known over the years with whom you've lost contact. In order to build and strengthen our relationships with others we must spend time with the important people in our lives engaging in frequent, open, honest, and kind communication.

Thus far I've talked a lot about nurturing your relationships, but every once in a while it's worth taking a hard look at these relationships and evaluating whether or not they are meeting your needs for love, friendship, and intimacy. Do you feel loved and accepted for who you really are? Do you feel a positive personal connection? Do you feel supported by your family members, friends, and loved ones? If you can honestly answer yes to these questions, then you are very blessed to be a part of such loving and supportive relationships. However, what if you are in a relationship that isn't making you feel loved and appreciated, that isn't supporting you and giving you what you need? If this is true for you, you know in your heart what you need to do. Deep down inside you know, but you just may be afraid to follow your heart. You may need to find the courage to distance yourself from the people who are making you feel unloved or less than. In extreme cases, it may be necessary to completely sever the relationship in order to ensure your physical, mental, and emotional well-being. Then you'll be free to establish new relationships with others that will truly nurture you and help you grow into the person that you were created to be.

Acceptance and Self-Love

Loving and accepting yourself is just as important, and perhaps more so, as establishing supportive relationships, because it boils down to this: you need to live with yourself for a very long time so you might as well make the most of it. Unfortunately so many of us go through life "under the influence" of negative thoughts derived from harsh words directed at us by trusted adults, difficult and emotionally charged circumstances, or unfavorable comparisons with others that occurred during our childhood years. Allow me to clarify this by saying that as young children who have not yet developed our own sense of self, we can easily internalize negative comments and emotions and spend the rest of our lives falsely believing in our perceived inadequacies. Our beliefs then turn into self-fulfilling prophecies, holding us back and limiting our opportunities in life. In looking back on my own life, I can easily see how the negative opinions that I harbored about myself and my abilities kept me from realizing my dream of becoming a teacher for many years. It was not until I was in my thirties and raising my own children that I finally challenged my long-held beliefs and successfully went back to school and became a teacher.

Tips for Self-Love and Acceptance:

- List five talents that you possess.
- Refrain from comparing yourself to others.
- Forgive yourself for past mistakes.
- List all the traits that you appreciate about yourself.
- Focus on the positive aspects of yourself.

While it is absolutely essential for your health and happiness that you love and accept yourself exactly as you are at this moment, I would encourage you to challenge some of the negative beliefs about yourself that may have been unwittingly planted during your childhood. When you do this you may find, as I did, that those limiting beliefs are not justified and can therefore be cast aside, giving you greater confidence and freedom to pursue your dreams. Further, as you gain greater knowledge and awareness of who you really are at your core, you can work toward acceptance and self-love by replacing those long-held negative thoughts with positive affirming thoughts. In accomplishing this task I've found mantras to be extremely useful in helping me to retrain my thoughts. A mantra is simply a sound, word, or phrase that is repeated over and over again to help focus your mind while you meditate. Feel free to experiment with the mantras that speak to your heart as you move forward on your healing journey.

> **Mantras for Self-Love:**
>
> **Acceptance:** I am an amazing creation and my best is good enough.
>
> **Respect:** I deserve to be happy and I follow my heart.
>
> **Awareness:** I am free to see what's inside of me.
>
> **Knowledge:** I know my heart and soul. This knowledge supports me and guides all I do.
>
> **Trust:** Less control brings me greater freedom and happiness.

Religion and Spirituality

Let me begin by saying that I feel blessed to live in the United States of America whose citizens are free to practice the religion of their choice. The founders of our country showed great wisdom in delineating freedom of religion as a basic civil right in the Bill of Rights. Before we go any further in discussing religion and spirituality, let's get clear on the terminology. According to the Merriam-Webster Dictionary religion has several definitions, the most pertinent ones for our discussion here being: "the service and worship of God or the supernatural" and "a personal set or institutionalized system of religious attitudes, beliefs, and practices".[15] However, while many people associate themselves with some form of religion or religious institution, an increasing number of people are distancing themselves from traditional organized religions, focusing instead on practicing their own personal forms of spirituality. Spirituality is defined as "sensitivity or attachment to religious values" and "the quality or state of being spiritual".[16] As this definition suggests religion and spirituality are closely related to one another, but spirituality is a distinct and separate concept. Spirituality gives the individual autonomy over his or her interpretation of the soul or spirit, whereas religion implies participation in a communal practice and interpretation of divine beliefs and worship. Bearing these differences in mind, before we can engage in any meaningful conversations around the subject of religion and spirituality, it is absolutely crucial that we respect and appreciate the varied religious beliefs and traditions followed by people across the country and around the world, particularly given the politically-charged world that we live in today.

It is in this spirit of mutual respect and understanding that you and I can come together with open hearts and minds to explore the benefits of cultivating strong spiritual connections. I'll start this conversation the only way I know how, by sharing my core religious beliefs on which my Christian faith is based. First and foremost, I believe in God, the creator of all, His son Jesus Christ, our Lord and Savior, and the spirit of God, the Holy Spirit at work in the world today. I further believe that God created all human beings in His image and likeness. Therefore, in addition to possessing a mind and body, all people have a spirit, often referred to as a "soul" in religious circles. The human spirit or soul is that special part of us that most closely reflects God's image. However, our spirit, being the invisible, innermost aspect of ourselves, can easily be neglected.

I'd like to share a little analogy here to emphasize the importance of nurturing our spirit. Having grown up in a family surrounded by mechanics, I can't help but liken the aspects of our human design to a car. A modern car today consists of several key components, three of which I'll focus on here. First, there is the body of the car, that which you can easily see and recognize, just like our own human body. Then there is the computer in the car that monitors and reports the car's performance, similar to the workings of the human mind. Lastly, and most importantly, there is the engine, which is responsible for powering the car. Our human spirit can be likened to the engine of the car in that it is the source or our inner strength and power.

Our spirit plays a vitally important role in our lives. It serves as our guide, helping us to more clearly discern what's true for us in our present circumstances and take necessary and appropriate actions in our lives. Our spirit gives us courage, strength, wisdom, and understanding and helps us to love others more perfectly, like God loves us. It is our human spirit that helps us to persevere, and for those blessed with the gift of faith, our faith in a good and loving God gives us comfort and hope during difficult or uncertain times in our lives.

Taking time to nurture our faith and our spirit has tremendous benefits, many of which often go unrecognized. However, just as physical exercise strengthens our body, spiritual exercise strengthens us spiritually, better preparing us to weather the storms of life and allowing us to make better, more insightful decisions in our daily lives. So as we can see, our human spirit is well worth nurturing in order that we can continue to enjoy the inner wisdom and strength that it imparts to us.

Tips to Nurture Spirituality:

- Spend 5-10 minutes each day in meditation or quiet prayer.
- Read and reflect on a Scripture passage from the Bible each day.
- Read an uplifting spiritual book.
- Perform a random act of kindness for someone.
- Take a class to learn more about your religion.
- Read about the lives and works of holy people or powerful spiritual leaders from the past.
- Go on a spiritual retreat.
- Join a Bible Study or small church community group.

Social Life

Having a healthy, balanced social life is also tremendously important for your overall health and wellness. Not only is an active social life a great way to stay connected to family and friends, but it is also a wonderful way to meet new people and expand you network of friends. However, it's not uncommon to hear someone say that they don't have time for a social life. Does this describe you?

Take a minute to assess your current social life. Are you taking the time each week to engage with others in activities that you enjoy or are you stuck in "work mode?" I was most definitely stuck in work mode for many years and didn't take much time to play and enjoy life. On my healing journey I came to understand just how imbalanced my life had become. I had to acknowledge that as my health had declined over the years I spent less and less time with family and friends, isolating myself to some extent. While I can look back and justify my lack of social interactions by claiming that I was too tired and caught up in the health challenges that I was facing, the fact remains that this way of living was not supporting my health and happiness, and I needed to make some serious changes.

Perhaps the most important change I made was centered on my mindset. Being a classic Type A personality and eternal perfectionist, I had been so focused on working to heal my health concerns that I had lost sight of the big picture. Eventually I came to the realization that I couldn't do this alone. This thought came to me so vividly when an acupuncturist whom I had been working with asked me, " Why don't you let the universe help you?" My whole perspective changed in that moment and from that point on I made a conscious effort to let my family and friends support me on my healing journey. Interestingly, but not surprisingly, when I reconnected with my family and friends and started reengaging in social activities with them, I began to feel happier, more energized and alive, in spite of my health concerns at the time, providing further proof of the power of cultivating strong social connections.

Tips for Nourishing a Balanced Social Life:

- Identify your passions and connect with groups or organizations that share your passions.
- Schedule a social activity with friends or family each week.
- Be open to new experiences.
- Volunteer your time once a month for a worthwhile cause that you believe in.
- Be as flexible with your schedule as possible.
- Engage in conversation with new people that you come in contact with.

Blue Zones

If you have any doubts about the power of having strong social and spiritual connections, look no further for proof than your nearest "Blue Zone." Blue Zones are geographical areas around the world whose populations enjoy the longest life spans on earth. From the five Blue Zones that have been identified, scientists and other researchers have determined the healthy lifestyle habits that appear to support increased longevity. Of the nine healthy lifestyle habits shared by these groups, three of them, accounting for more than thirty percent of the total, are grounded in a combination of social and spiritual connections.[17] In light of this fact, the Blue Zones are a true testament to the power of strong social and spiritual connections in helping people to live longer, happier, and healthier lives.

10

Powerful Resources to Support You

"I've learned that fear limits your vision. It serves as blinders to what may be just a few steps down the road for you. The journey is valuable, but believing in your talents, your abilities, and your self-worth can empower you to walk down an even brighter path. Transforming fear into freedom – how great is that?"

Soledad O'Brien

Allergies and Food Sensitivities:

- ***The Allergy Solution: Unlock the Surprising, Hidden Truth about Why You Are Sick and How to Get Well,*** book by Leo Galland, M.D. and Jonathan Galland, J.D. (New York: Hay House, Inc., 2016)

  This book contains valuable information and

insights about allergies and provides action steps to address allergies.

- ***Gluten Free and More Magazine* (Norwalk, CT: Belvoir Media Group, LLC)**

    This magazine is for people with celiac disease, food allergies, and food sensitivities. It contains helpful product reviews and lifestyle tips, current medical information, and easy allergy-free recipes.

Autoimmune Disease:

- ***The Autoimmune Solution: Prevent and Reverse the Full Spectrum of Inflammatory Symptoms and Diseases,* book by Amy Myers, M.D. (New York: HarperCollins, 2015)**
- ***Eat Dirt: Why Leaky Gut May Be the Root Cause of Your Health Problems and 5 Surprising Steps to Cure It,* book by Dr. Josh Axe (New York: HarperCollins, 2016)**
- ***The Autoimmune Fix: How to Stop the Hidden Autoimmune Damage that Keeps You Sick, Fat, and Tired Before It Turns into Disease,* book by Tom O'Bryan, DC, CCN, DACBN (New York: Rodale, 2016)**

    These books were written by functional medicine doctors who share a wealth of scientific information about factors relating to autoimmune disease and offer medical advice from a functional medicine perspective as well as recipes to support healing.

Blue Zones:

- *www.bluezones.com/2016/11/power-9/*
  On this website you'll learn about the nine healthy lifestyle habits shared by the world's longest living people and access related articles and recipes.

Breathing Exercises:

- **Mindful Breathing Exercises:** *www.drweil.com/ health-wellness/body-mind-spirit/stress-anxiety/ breathing-three-exercises/*
  This website showcases three mindful breathing exercises to help reduce stress and promote relaxation.

Doctor Directories:

- **Functional Medicine Doctors:**
  - **Institute for Functional Medicine Referral Network:** *www.ifm.org/ find-a-practitioner/*
- **Integrative Medicine Doctors:**
  - **Academy of Integrative Health and Medicine:** *www.aihm.org/search/ custom.asp?id=4620*
  - **The University of Arizona Center for Integrative Medicine:** *www. integrativemedicine.arizona.edu/ alumni.html*

- **Naturopathic Doctors:**
  - **Directory of American Association of Naturopathic Physicians:** *www.naturopathic.org/ AF_MemberDirectory.asp*

  These websites gives you access to online directories to help you find a doctor near you.

Environmental Health Information:

- **Environmental Working Group (EWG):** *www. ewg.org*

  This website gives you access to the latest research and information about issues affecting public health and the environment.
- **EWG's Annual Shoppers Guide to Pesticides in Produce:** *www.ewg.org/foodnews*

  This website gives you access to the most current version of the **Clean Fifteen** and **Dirty Dozen** lists.

Exercise:

- **Online Workouts:** *makeyourbodywork.com/ how-to-exercise-at-home/*

  This website gives you access to fifty free online workouts that teach you how to work out safely and efficiently at home.

Fermenting:

- **Fermenting Products:** *www. nourishedessentials.com*

  This website is the home of **The Easy Fermenter** line of fermenting products and offers free fermenting tips, recipes, and instructional videos on fermenting.

Food:

- **Thrive Market:** *www.thrivemarket.com*

  This is an online market that offers a wide variety of natural and organic products at discounted prices.

- ***The Autoimmune Solution Cookbook: Over 150 Delicious Recipes to Prevent and Reverse the Full Spectrum of Inflammatory Symptoms and Diseases,* book by Amy Myers, M.D. (New York: HarperCollins, 2018)**

  This cookbook is full of Autoimmune Protocol Diet (AIP) recipes.

- ***It's All Good: Delicious, Easy Recipes that Will Make You Look Good and Feel Great,* book by Gwyneth Paltrow and Julia Turshen (New York: Grand Central Life and Style, 2013)**

  This cookbook does not contain AIP-specific recipes but it has a variety of Elimination Diet, vegan, and protein-packed recipes to try.

- ***Against All Grain: Delectable Paleo Recipes to Eat Well and Feel Great,* book by Daniel Walker (Las Vegas: Victory Belt Publishing, 2013)**

- *Against All Grain: Meals Made Simple: Gluten-Free, Dairy-Free, and Paleo Recipes to Make Anytime,* book by Daniel Walker (Las Vegas: Victory Belt Publishing, 2014)

  Danielle Walker's *Against All Grain* cookbooks do not contain AIP-specific recipes but they are full of gluten-free, grain-free, and dairy-free recipes, which I'm sure you'll enjoy.

- *The Whole30: The 30-Day Guide to Total Health and Food Freedom,* book by Melissa Hartwig and Dallas Hartwig (New York: Houghton Mifflin Harcourt, 2015)

- *The Whole30 Cookbook: 150 Delicious and Totally Compliant Recipes to Help You Succeed with the Whole30 and Beyond,* book by Melissa Hartwig (New York: Houghton Mifflin Harcourt, 2016)

  The Whole30[R] is an elimination diet program and these books contain many delicious anti-inflammatory recipes and a wealth of information to help you enjoy a healthier body and develop a healthier relationship with food in the process.

Grounding:

- **Commercial Grounding Systems:** *www.earthing.com*

  This site has information about grounding and sells a variety of personal grounding products.

Healthy Living:

- ***The Urban Monk: Eastern Wisdom and Modern Hacks to Stop Time and Find Success, Happiness, and Peace*, book by Pedram Shojai, OMD (New York: Rodale, 2016)**
  This book contains practical advice and resources to help you to live a healthier and happier life.
- ***Sharecare*, app developed by Sharecare, Inc.**
  This free health and fitness app allows you to track your health and habits, and it offers a whole library of health information to support positive lifestyle changes.

Meditations:

- ***Insight Timer*, app developed by Insight Network Inc.**
  This free app has a large library of over 10,000 meditations.

Mindfulness and Personal Choices:

- ***The Secret*, book by Rhonda Byrne (New York: Atria Books/Beyond Words Publishing, 2006)**
  This book explores the power of our thoughts in manifesting things in our lives.

- ***Resisting Happiness,*** **book by Matthew Kelly (New York: Beacon Publishing, 2016)**

  This book guides us on a personal dive into the choices that we make in our everyday lives.

Relationships:

- ***30 Days to Taming Your Tongue: What You SAY (and DON'T SAY) Will Improve Your Relationships,*** **book by Deborah Smith Pegues (Eugene, Oregon: Harvest House Publishers, 2005)**

  This book explores many of the negative ways that we communicate with others, leading us to a greater awareness and encouraging us to move beyond our negative communication patterns.

Religion and Spirituality:

- ***Everything Starts from Prayer: Mother Teresa's Meditations on Spiritual Life for People of All Faiths,*** **book by Anthony Stern, M.D. (Ashland, Oregon: White Cloud Press, 2009)**

  Mother Teresa was a profoundly holy woman and spiritual leader in her own right, and this book is full of her words of wisdom on prayer and spirituality.

Sleep:

- ***Pillow,*** **app developed by Neybox Digital Ltd.**
  This free app tracks the quantity and quality of your sleep using an Apple Watch or an iPhone or iPad placed close to your pillow.

Citations

Chapter 2

1. Campos, Marcelo. "Leaky Gut: What Is It, and What Does It Mean for You?" *Harvard Health Blog*, Harvard Health Publishing, 21 Sept. 2017, www.health.harvard.edu/blog/leaky-gut-what-is-it-and-what-does-it-mean-for-you-2017092212451. Web. 26 June 2018.
2. Campos, Marcelo. "Leaky Gut: What Is It, and What Does It Mean for You?" *Harvard Health Blog*, Harvard Health Publishing, 21 Sept. 2017, www.health.harvard.edu/blog/leaky-gut-what-is-it-and-what-does-it-mean-for-you-2017092212451. Web. 26 June 2018.
3. School, Harvard Medical. "Inflammation: A Unifying Theory of Disease - Harvard Health." *Harvard Health Blog*, Harvard Health Publishing, Apr. 2006, www.health.harvard.edu/newsletter_article/Inflammation_A_unifying_theory_of_disease. Web. 27 June 2018.

Chapter 4

4. Fletcher, Jenna. "Anti-Inflammatory Diet: Food List and Tips." Reviewed by Natalie Butler, *Medical News Today*, MediLexicon

International, 3 Dec. 2017, www.medicalnewstoday.com/articles/320233. Web. 4 July 2018

5.   Macmillan, Amanda. "Non-Celiac Wheat Sensitivity Is Real and Linked to Leaky Gut, Study Says." *Health.com*, Health Magazine, 28 July 2016, www.health.com/digestive-health/leaky-gut-wheat-sensitivity. Web. 6 July 2018

6.   Burgess, Lana. "AIP Diet: What Is It and What Can You Eat?" Reviewed by Natalie Butler, *Medical News Today*, MediLexicon International, 30 Nov. 2017, www.medicalnewstoday.com/articles/320195.php. Web. 6 July 2018

Chapter 6

7.   National Research Council (US) Committee on Drug Use in Food Animals. The Use of Drugs in Food Animals: Benefits and Risks. Washington (DC): National Academies Press (US); 1999. 2, Food-Animal Production Practices and Drug Use https://www.ncbi.nlm.nih.gov/books/NBK232573/. Web. 2 Aug. 2018

8.   Peachman, Rachel Rabkin. "What's Really in Your Meat?" *Consumer Reports*, Oct. 2018, pp. 30–37.

9.   Bottemiller, Helena. "Dispute over Drug in Feed Limiting US Meat Exports." *NBCNews.com*, NBCUniversal News Group, 25 Jan. 2012, www.nbcnews.com/business/markets/dispute-over-drug-feed-limiting-us-meat-exports-flna174014. Web. 2 Aug. 2018

10. Coyle, Daisy. "8 Surprising Things That Harm Your Gut Bacteria." *Healthline*, Healthline Media, 19 June 2017, www.healthline.com/nutrition/8-things-that-harm-gut-bacteria. Web. 2 Sept. 2018

Chapter 7

11. Oschman, James L, Gaétan Chevalier, and Richard Brown. "The Effects of Grounding (earthing) on Inflammation, the Immune Response, Wound Healing, and Prevention and Treatment of Chronic Inflammatory and Autoimmune Diseases." *Journal of Inflammation Research* 8 (2015): 83–96. *PMC*. www.ncbi.nlm. nih.gov/pmc/articles/PMC4378297/. Web. 30 July 2018.

Chapter 8

12. Crosta, Peter. "Insomnia: Causes, Symptoms, and Treatments." *Medical News Today*, MediLexicon International, 7 Dec. 2017, www.medicalnewstoday.com/articles/9155.php. Web. 1 Aug. 2018

13. Semeco, Arlene. "The Top 10 Benefits of Regular Exercise." *Healthline*, Healthline Media, 10 Feb. 2017, www.healthline. com/nutrition/10-benefits-of-exercise. Web. 2 Aug. 2018

Chapter 9

14. McLeod, S. A. "Maslow's Hierarchy of Needs." *Simply Psychology*, Simply Psychology, 21 May 2018, www.simplypsychology.org/ maslow.html. Web. 3 Sept. 2018

15. "Religion." *Merriam-Webster*, Merriam-Webster, www.merriam-webster.com/dictionary/religion. Web. 9 Sept. 2018.

16. "Spirituality." *Merriam-Webster*, Merriam-Webster, www. merriam-webster.com/dictionary/spirituality. Web. 9 Sept. 2018.

17. Buettner, Dan. "Power 9®." *Blue Zones*, Blue Zones, LLC, 27 Dec. 2017, www.bluezones.com/2016/11/power-9/. Web. 16 Sept. 2018

Meet the Author

Mary Ann Camarillo

After struggling with mysterious autoimmune symptoms for over ten years, Mary Ann decided to take her health into her own hands and embarked on her own healing journey. She experimented with alternative medical therapies and dedicated herself to learning all she could about autoimmune disease and its root causes.

Eventually her journey brought her to the Institute for Integrative Nutrition where Mary Ann gained further knowledge about healthy diet and lifestyle choices while studying to be an Integrative Nutrition Health Coach. Since resolving her own chronic health issues, Mary Ann is passionate about helping others overcome autoimmune or other chronic conditions so they too can enjoy greater health and happiness.

Notes

Notes

Notes

Notes

Notes

Notes

Notes

Notes

Notes

Notes